Do You Want

Your Brain

to Hurt

Now or Later?

Judi Kaufman

Bombshelter Press

Los Angeles / 2007

ISBN: 0-941017-80-x

Bombshelter Press
www.bombshelterpress.com
books@bombshelterpress.com
PO Box 481266 Bicentennial Station
Los Angeles, California 90048 USA

Printed in the United States of America

Ftont cover art: Lisa Jane Persky, *Psychpart*

Layout & design: Alan Berman

Art of the Brain Logo: Kim Baer–KBDA Inc

There's no way to thank everyone who has supported me in my life and in my art. Each of you in your own special way has helped me overcome obstacles and move on. The greatest blessing in my life is that it would take a book to list all those friends and loved ones who have been there for me, helping me to take another day with love and gratitude. I am truly blessed. Many of the poems in this book were first shared with my writing buddies in the Los Angeles Poets and Writers Collective, and I want to thank them for their encouragement and enthusiasm. Each day is a feast, and I thank all of you, everyone, for the goodies set upon the table.

Richard Arthurs
(read the poem "Seven Cards")

Bobbi Asimow,
who taught me how to die

James Lee Barrett,
the person who taught me to understand great writing

Klaus Barth,
an ironman and a true man of iron

Hermione Brown
my mentor as a human being

Louis Brown,
a friend who urged me forward

Marilyn Fortner,
painter and friend

Harriet Goldberg,
a woman I know through the memories of her husband, Victor

Gerry Haims,
who was a bowl of cherries

Lucy Herscher,
a mother and grandmother with two sons who are rabbis

Stanley Josephs,
doctor, poet, humanitarian

Fred Kaufman,
my brother-in-law who lived his life his way

Ericia Lohrer Knapp,
whose son Patrick told me the heart of the family was ripped out when his mother passed away

George and Rhoda Krone,
who made great parents for Steve, Neil, and Ruth

Ben Lautman—
I wish I had met him

Shari Lewis,
a class act who brought joy to children of all ages

Robert W. Morgan,
who used his truth as a way to instill wisdom, thought and values

Christopher Penn,
who taught me how to love

Leo Penn,
an actor, director, father and a gentle man

Christopher Schmitz,
a beautiful boy who was a man before his time

Eleanor and Sam Stone,
a couple who believed in making love after funerals

Michael Tarr,
who remained true to himself

Tony Trattner,
a man for all seasons

Simon Wolen,
who loved his daughter's values and creativity

Payson Wolff,
a man of integrity, high fashion, and the law

You are all part of my heart and brain. You helped me to appreciate what humanness is. Your individuality inspires my own. You light my path.
With my love and gratitude,
Judi

. . . and to the men and women
who have fought
and are fighting
for freedom all over the world

Acknowledgments

I'd like to acknowledge the following friends and fellow artists, some of whom have read various versions of these poems during the editing of this book and offered valuable suggestions and insights.

Darya Allen-Attar

Dean Ambrose and Sally Cole

Richard Dean Anderson and his daughter Wylie

Lynn and Brian Arthurs

Michael Asimow and Family

Bobbi Asimow

Shula Bahat

Maxine and Arthur Barens

Merete Barrett

Michael and Karen Berk

Howard Bernstein and Bunny Wasser

Mitchell Bloch

Mark and Patty Borden

Harold and Ruth Borden

Howy and Cedar Boschan

Paul and Grace Boschan

Robert and Bobbie Boschan

Leonie Brandstetter

Michael and Elaine Bridge

Dr. Jill Broffman

Joyce and Bill Bromiley

Marcia Burnam

Rod and Sandra Campbell

Cat, Scott, Caylin, and Kaya Cannady

Monica Cantor

David and Marlene Capell

Robert and Jan Carusi

Chiwan Choi

Douglas, Jennifer and Chloe Chu

John and Dr. Beverly Chu

Jonathan Chu

Bruce and Christine Churchill and their twins John Barrett and Wylie Suyin Churchill

Laralee Ciernia

Maureen Clavin

Dr. Timothy Cloughesy

Bruce and Toni Corwin

Dorothy Corwin

Joan and Gerald Doren

Clint and Dina Eastwood

Edward Egan

Mark and Lynn Egerman

Joan and William Feldman

Steve and Sarah Fortner

Bonnie Fuller

Richard Furman

Gang, Tyre, Ramer and Brown

Stanley and Ilene Gold

Jack, Lori, and Josh Grapes

Jill Greenwald

Jennifer Herrguth

Doris Haims

David Harris

Jacques Heims

Cashia Helleckson and family

Martha Henderson

Dick Henkel

Rabbi Uri and Dr. Myna Herscher

Nancy and Alan Jacobson

Fred and Margareta Jamner

Roy and Anne Jespersen

Maria Cristina Jimenez

Jim and Leslie Kaji

Paul and Sally Kanin

Leona and Ronald Katz

Jill and Aly Kaufman

Donna and Les Kaufman

Roy, Jennifer and Suzy Kaufman

Naz Kaykhosrowpour

Laura King

Patrick Knapp

Steve Krone, Heidi Rummel, and
their children Jonathan, Charlotte,
and Annie Rose

Dan and Joann Lautman

Ruth Lavine

Duane Law

Patti Lawhon

Jean Lee

Jamie Levine and Dr. Karen
Rashcovsky

Mark and Cathy Loucheim

Paula and Sidney Machtinger

Bert and Phyllis Massing

Joe and Justine Medeiros

Jeffrey and Kim Nemoy

Benedicta and Geoff Oblath

John and Margaret Ord

Eileen Penn

Pituitary Network Association

Steve and Sandy Polin

Ann Ramer

Bruce and Madeline Ramer

Gregg Ramer

Neal and Jeannine Ramer and their
son Eli

Marc and Tira Ramer, their son
Jacob, and their daughter Mayah

Nancy Rishagen

Glynis Robert

Herb and Joyce Rosenblum

David and Lori Rousso

Ken and Wendy Ruby

Nady and Debbie Saidoff

William Sater and Elise Sinay

Cookie Shapiro

Mace Siegel

Barbara Silberbusch

Steven and Gale Sills

Jerry and Sharon Simon

Arnold and Rachel Smith

Kenny Smith

Fred and Susie Stern

Jerry and Stephanie Stern

John Stewart and Michael Nourse

Alexandra and Jordan Sussman

Karl and DeeDee Sussman

Tamara Taback

Janice Tarr

Ted and Carolyn Tyler

Len and Cathy Unger

Gy and Jadi Waldron

Dennis and Ruth Wasser

Lew and Dale Weitzman

Sherry Wertenbruch

Pam Whitham

Adele and Irwin Wiener

Dr. John Winters

Adele Yellin

Dr. Jacob Zighelboim

Contents

Hi
high
Hello
Come on into my home, my brain
Watch out, I am going to give you a hug
Chai
I want to give you a hug
I am a hugger
It is the way I speak
My hugs are clear and big and hard
Since my second brain surgery
I speak with a slur or a lisp
a verbal limp
so, welcome to my favorite words
Some of them are Hebrew or Yiddish
Like *chai*
high
Words that come
When I listen to my memories
Stay tuned to
the glory of brain cancer
It has been good for me
I have found me
In me
Layer by layer
For me.
As I look into light and gray matter
Words I want to speak
Life, *chai*
go inside to the loss
Of words
Please celebrate for me.

These bright days are not about perfect brains.
They are about imperfections.
Flaws and tears.
Fears, painting, the art of painting pain!
Sharing parents.
Flaws.
My friend said his baby wasn't born perfect!
None of us were born perfect.
Days are brighter as we share our imperfections,
our fears, our flaws, our pain.
Perfection is not about real human beings.
Perfection is a cartoon, without the humor.
Perfection cuts away the core of caring.
Perfection is a hidden illness.

2005 has turned Art of the Brain into Art of the International Heart of Brain Injury for me. From the tsunami, hemispheres away, to our geography, America in Louisiana. People have survived the giant wave and Hurricane Katrina.

I have survived two brain cancer surgeries. Our brains' hemispheres are not insured for survival. Pssst, we are all brain-injured. Terrified. The gulf coasts, the Arabian Sea, and the Bay of Bengal are a collection of massive malignant brain tumors. Tumors of terror.

From Israel and Iraq, we are all terrified. We are changed. We are all brain-injured from change. G-d and nature change things.

We learn to survive. To appreciate sunlight, and the light our own brains give off. Trees that continue to grow, even when half-drowned by the dark water of tsunamis and hurricanes.

My family and friends have been changed by so many kinds of terror. I welcome their change and all their many colors. We are here to help each other to survive the terror and the change that comes after.

Pssssst, G-d. What are you doing, bud? I was thinking about you. You know I like you, G-d. I thought about getting together for a drink or something. But I don't drink. I would like to go to a circus. I want to have fun. Take care of myself. You know, G-d, I am in the hot seat. I have to get my affairs in order. Durable power of attorney, and all that, I need a witness I can trust with my truth. There are a bunch of boxes to check, that's easy. But pink cotton candy and a red snow cone? Where am I gonna get that? Let's use a feather duster with a handle to dust off the old clowns. Will you buy me a balloon? You can pick the color.

Yep, G-d, I have been trying to talk to you for a long time. You don't hear me, G-d. You want to be the big cheese. Take charge. Now I have the right to give instructions about my care. Come on in to my circus tent full of animals and urges. G-d, I have been reading your big book. There is a lot of stuff in there about passion. My favorite subject. I think about passion all the time. You know, G-d, it is time for you to add a new chapter to your work. All the stuff about the 10 Commandments, Job. Adam. Eve. Abraham. Isaac. Moses. Jacob. It's good stuff. It's hopeful. But, right now, you need to listen to me. G-d! You didn't accentuate passion enough. Just add a chapter. What's the big deal?

You know, G-d, passion both enhances and erodes character. Exultation, Risk. Adventure. You seem to want me to be in the center ring with a balancing act. But life can never be in balance. When I like or love people, I need to be connected to their character, their chatter. When I am not. Life....or as you would call it, *Chai*, G-d, is thrown out of kilter.

So, G-d, can you listen for a minute? Don't interrupt. Laugh or cry. I like it when you show me who your really are. Listen, G-d. I need you. I told you I don't want to be useless, a vegetable. I don't want to settle for selfishness. The right thing, according to your book, is to choose life. I choose life. I love life. Life with family, friends, but not a life that intrudes on spirit. So, G-d, please add a paragraph in your testament about me. I know that this is asking a lot. You have so many people asking for your help. I understand. I have always understood. I'll keep it short.

Please refuse consent to keep me alive if I am a pole holding up the circus tent. Please fire docs or directors that think I need to stay alive to do a half-assed job of fund-raising. Please disapprove of procedures that eliminate my passion. You are my agent, G-d. I haven't limited your authority. I have given you supreme power to be all of who you are with all your greatness and gifts. G-d. I am a wife, mother, friend. I am an artist, a fund-raiser. You are smart. I trust you, G-d. Please make the right choice, the choice that you would make for yourself. I like you, G-d. Thanks for everything. Remember, my brain surgery is next week, June 12th, 2003 at UCLA. Come visit me.

Have you heard that Judi Kaufman is brain-injured?
She has taken up religion.
Judi-ism is supposed to get her through life.
Poor Roy.
Now, that Judi is full of herself.
I liked her better as a prude.
Poor Roy.
She has turned into a funny flirt.
Old wives' tales have taken their toll.
Yep, you got that right: she is cock-eyed.

I like Ben Franklin. I began to think more about him watching his biography on KCET. He founded the first public library. He was an inventor. I wanted to be an inventor. Imagine his brain! Its bright light. Bifocals! The lightning rod! The odometer! The wood stove! Ben. Benjamin Franklin. A Founding Father, The kind of father I wanted. A man of nuance. *Poor Richard's Almanac*. His frank brain. His founding-father mentality. Moving me to open my mind.

I have been thinking about books on Ben. Since I like Ben, I want something more from him. "You have a vivid imagination," Roy says, rubbing his thumb against his lip. He agreed with my neuro-oncologist. "You can't be a CEO. Those skills were removed from your right frontal lobe along with your brain tumor. "You are a CAO. Corporate Artistic Officer." Passion drained by truth. Dry-eye logic. "But, Judi," he said, you have never been logical. "I'm your CEO. You're my CAO," he said.

Corporate Artistic Officer. I like that. I have been sculpting pedestals for years. Pedestals for people with high IQs and talents I don't have. Recovering from brain cancer, I had no IQ. I couldn't find my way home. I didn't recognize a calendar. Sex was the only thing in my mind. I watched close friends leave their mates. They found the fun of a fresh body. Juicy ideas. Me, I was missing. Roy was looking for me, the me that had CEO skills, social skills, some sex skills, words. Three male friends found three delicious females. I put the three couples on a pedestal. Front and center. Seductive.

Roy was front and center in my recovery. He turned off the lights and the heat. He counted pills. He hid his terror. He tried to cure me. He bought a Palm Pilot. He knew how to hot sync it to his hard drive. He knew where I should be. He went to every MRI appointment. He gave me his handkerchief when I began to have seizures. During the seizures, I was petrified I would die alone. Roy was always there when I woke up.

I put the three couples under a magnifying glass. I wanted to find the secret to passion and give it to Roy. He used to say, early in our relationship, "I can't stand to see sickness and suffering." During movies like *My Left Foot* and *Lorenzo's Oil*, he left the theater. He couldn't stand to see it. Yet all through my diagnosis, the surgery, the recovery, the seizures that come and go, he has been there when I woke up. He's always there when I wake up, the witness to my suffering, the vessel of my passions, holding my love.

The good news is
I have invented a new Bacterium for all the other things
that are wrong with me.
I know the back door to the cafeteria where
so many bacteria live and breathe.
I am finally the opposite of being out "I AM IN, I AM IN!"
I got sick at the airport,
And they told me I had a terminal illness.
I am proud to say that my pelvis is a second cousin to Elvis.
The medical staff gave me a cane, so I could walk
to a good room for hiding.
The room is called secretion.
In Secretion I have tons of tablets.
Come on, you know what they are: small tables.
They transferred me to the recovery room,
a place to redo my upholstery,
you know, my sweetie, my skin and fins.
The good news is that I am Di-lated,
I will live long.
I think I want to move to the Caesarean section of Rome
to get away from my enema.

I strut, chest out,
since my yoga trainer told me,
"Put your shoulders on your back."
I was clueless, believe me,
What the hell does it mean?
Put your shoulders on your back!
I have no idea
what a lot of words mean.
My physical therapist said,
"Hey Jud, no disclaimers about yourself are allowed."
Keep educating yourself.
Realize you're on your own
and you will know
the meaning of "autodidact."
"But, Dr. Gitlin," I tell my psychopharmacologist,
I am brain dead so much of the time."
I need a whole new education.
My friend said I belong in a VIP brain room.
Only certain people and information pass through the blood-brain barrier.
I learn a whole new set of words every day.
Dammitol, take two
and the rest of the world can go to hell
for up to eight full hours.

I smell things that others can't smell.
I smell body odor and halitosis.
Is it the lack of brushing
or fussing with a shower?
Odors attack me from the eastern star,
western sunset, North Pole.
Not to mention the shit on southwestern boots.
I recently learned that my hypersensitivity to smell
is a result of the two golf balls cut out of my brain!
I got some serious issues.
Are friends and family fair game?
Do I follow the truth to the far end of the fairway?
Or do I just stop breathing?

I am getting *sick* from Cliché,
I may even die from it.
So I am going to switch over to palindromes.
Palin equals again plus *drom* equals run.
(palin=AGAIN + drom, draime=RUN)
I'm running around like a chicken with my head cut off.
(Oops! another cliché.)
A palindrome is a word or phrase which reads the same in both directions.
When I die I want to die from a P-word.
I want to pop with passion.
Not from a C-word, like *Cliché*.
If I die from Passion, I will be an EYE, a DEED,
a PIP, RADAR, or a TOOT.
A RACECAR.
A REDIVIDER,
the longest single English word in common usage that is a palindrome.
I'll be a Redivider, separating me from death.

A verb is exactly what I want to be.
A class of words expressing action.
And existence.
Or occurrence.
I am the main part of a predicate.

For 24 seasons the lights in the stadium have been on my baseball cap.
All the players of hardball have question marks on their caps and foreheads.
A "C" opened to the left with a dirty eye attached to its bottom.
Those dirty eyes; it changed into a hot dog with a dollop of mustard under
     the pitcher's mound.
My glove catches all the dirt from base sliding.
No, I mean from slippery speech.
I have gone into overtime looking for the national title for
     slow pitch soft ball.
My lips are bleeding from all the hours I have had to stand in the sun for
     day games.
The dot floats from person to person from player to player on a lace hankie.
Out of loyalty and love I have changed from an LA Dodger fan into a New
     York Yankee fan.
I ask myself, What do I look like when I strike out?
I am scratching and adjusting my missing soft balls.
"Hey, G-d, turn your lights down, it's making me squint and starve for
     success."
I don't recognize when I hit a homer and fans are yelling,
     "Way to go, Babe!"
Wow, when I hit my ball out of the park, I'm on the front page,
Not in the bleachers where I am lost and just a number and looking for real
     food, not a hotdog.

Mommy, oh Mommy, *Oy gevalt, oy gevalt, oy gevalt.* My brain won't stop. My brain won't stop roaring. The chant becomes a tsunami, thousands of waves washing ashore. I welcome them into my cerebellum. A mass of walnuts, waving.

Using a piece of seaweed I pole vault from the middle of the ocean onto a stage of hexagons, pentagons, triangles and rectangles scattered across the sand dunes. I am not doomed. I see so much ahead. Congruent circles on a golden grid. *Feh!* It waves me on. "Cut the Yiddish," I roar.

Don't you dare infer that I am *drek.*

My mind swims with tropical fish from deep in the ocean. My mind is an aquarium of angular loss.

"Shooo! Splash!" My brain is a wave. *Oy vey, Oy gevalt.* The ocean holds tons of tuna. Seaweed accents every splash. I swim with the stingray. My brain is a tsunami.

It teaches me a new way to wave. "Hell. Sorry, I mean hello," I say.

Lo and behold, deep in the darkest water I see more, much more Non-Euclidian geometry.

An aquarium rises out of nowhere. Ocean swells, pregnant with new life.

A moonbeam enhances the golden grid. Perfectly defined.

Where did it come from, this gorgeous grid?

The mothering force has set me free from the shadows.

My heart is broken. Fart. A jellyfish carried away the stinky gas I passed when I swam ashore.

Shadows on some discarded whale. I wove it together as I have everything I ever knew about my mother and father.

People are so much bigger than the ocean. They are.

My shells.

My fish.

My salt from the sea.

Clam shells, mussels, separate water from sand from which I hear the roaring and the chanting of the ocean. Mother nature, my mommy.

Mother, I stutter like a flying fish. Help me, Mommy, I need to clear out the clutter.

Make me better. Then we can swim and say all the things we never said, because I stutter.

I wear a scaly T-shirt. It hurts.

Mothers simply forget because they are busy making jelly.

I have been stung. I am crying I need your skin to wipe my nose against. Or maybe your fins will work better.

I am sick of being sick over what happens to children without their mommies.

My sick brain.

Our true history
Is a wave in the ocean.
We will meet up.
We will meet up
With all those we have loved
Where light shines.

Holier than thou.
Her handwriting is illegible.
She sends tons of e-mails for thank you notes.
She has given up all those beautiful cards.
She talks baby talk.
Poor Judi.
She makes framed cards with dried-out rose petals.
Poor Judi.
She will never be the same.
She still plays dress up and wants to wear Mary Jane's.

G-d, I will not castrate him.
He doesn't have to tell me he is afraid.
The light in his eyes is gone.
His left eye droops.
He doesn't want to be in the spotlight.
Let this bypass keep him safe.

I have been in a relationship with calories since the day I was born.

Is a calorie a measure of heat or of hunger?

Hunger for food, for a menu of people,

I've eaten my heart out. I've dieted and saved myself for Sunday splurges.

My constant battle of the bulge.

My battle to draw people to me with my self discipline.

Or is it to touch people so they will touch me,

if only to whet their appetites.

For splurges I create menus to touch people.

Cheese fondue with red, yellow, and green-handled forks. No serving
        spoons, strictly served by hand so that touching's a must.

Sushi in passionate Asian restaurants is just what my doctor
        ordered for touching.

Colorful raw fish served on a beautiful naked woman.

Calories and colors are complicated.

I was excited, I found out that there are fish that change their gender
        depending on what's needed. When a male fish passes on or becomes
        weaker than the female fish, the strongest female fish becomes the
        new dominant male fish.

So now, I ask myself a new question: Am I a little fish in a little bowl?

And if so, a little sole or a little bass?

Or am I a big fish in a big bowl?

Am I in fresh water eager to be caught?

In a glass bowl waiting to be fed?

Am I male or female?

Strong or weak?

Am I a salmon swimming upstream?

Am I a Pacific Marlin with a long horn?

Or am I the naked woman on which they serve the colorful fish?

Heat. Hunger. Passion.

Sometimes I'm caught and thrown back. Sometimes I swim around hiding
        from the line.

Sometimes I have a shell.

Sometimes I'm eaten and feel myself being digested

And sometimes I just swim around and around. Alone.

A fat and sassy fish.

How sweet the cucumbers are this year.
It was an intimate gathering.
He can't see that I am growing.
I do great deeds.
I reach over to my night stand.
I gaze into the breath.
I hate assumptions.
Asshole.
Craveless.

The men I have loved remain in my mind like cells that won't be radiated away.

I still remember them, after two brain surgeries. Sometimes, I remember the good times. Not the times they walked away. I don't discard people who have loved me or liked me or even who have lied to me. I don't expect clever conversation. I just want someone I can talk to.

I egg on my ex's. I write to all of them. Maybe they'll respond. Maybe not. I don't care. Perhaps they don't care either.

Each of their shells contains core ingredients of who I once was and who I still am. I like the way they made me feel. I want to remain within ear range of their whispered jokes.

The smell of their shirts.

Their balls.

Their bravery.

Their saliva.

Their sadness.

Their truths.

Their lies.

Their lust.

I decide to send an email to all the men I have loved. Ben. Tricky Dickie. Roy! I have no idea what to say. I take a week, to find the right words. Even if my words are unclever, I will write to all of them. Maybe they'll respond, maybe not. I don't care. Perhaps they don't care either. Either way, I will have tried to say thank you for allowing me to love them.

I wear a bracelet that says HIGH-RISK PREGNANCY. My twins, the one growing in my brain and the one in my heart, have caused me to have all kinds of new labels.

First I was Judith, then I became Judy with a "Y."

In the fifth grade my sister said, "Spell your name with an 'I'! Be different."

Insinuate that you are different. There are too many Judys with a "Y." You don't want to be a multiple. Set fires.

Get out there, be bigger than life. My sister still says the same thing now that I have touched death twice. Now that I have an official label: BRAIN-INJURED! HIGH-RISK!

I continue to set fires. Matches sear my skin. I am like an onion, peeled away layer by layer.

I'm the fall guy.

Me. Mois. Judi with an "I." I am brain-injured.

Terrorized. Troubled by so much MUSH.

Nice.

But bitter.

Lonely.

When I have no reason to be lonely.

I am alive and I am married.

But I need to feel my loneliness. I need to know its meaning.

My pain must be felt in its own way.

I come from my yesterdays and when any one of them disappears, a part of me disappears too.

I'm trying to say "goodbye" in a good way, with gratitude. Then I can learn to hold on in a new way.

So I refuse to settle for sadness. I am proud to say, "I AM A NUT CASE."

I could care less about "I's" and "Y's." I am a walnut. I am encased in a shell that looks like my old brain.

I refuse to be a prefix.
I refuse to fix things that can't stand on their own.
I refuse to qualify or limit people, places or things.
I refuse to modify actions.
I will stand tall as an advertisement.
I am an advertisement for life.

I am obsessed with him and it has changed us all.
I laugh, sourly.
He keeps saying the same old thing.
I like you.
Alibis spoken into the microphone.
I stare at the wonder of the dagger.
I slip my hands inside his open shirt.

If I let my Art die
I will not survive.
So I take the ocean
Out of darkness.
Out of ego.
Out of the non-circle-idian.

Last week,
I was part of an ice sculpture.
That's right, baby, an ice sculpture,
a nude Eve.
Next to me was Adam, with the tip of his dick exposed,
looking just like a crabby apple.
Cell by cell, my skin flaked off,
exposing my geography.
The dam held back all of my water.
It was made of crabby apples,
cranberries, celery, spinach, squash,
tomatoes and *tamatos.*
Lo and behold, I was myself at 18,
a woman like Africa, half discovered,
half wild, with fertile soil.
At 30, I was like America,
well-developed and open to trade,
especially with men with a twinkle in their eye.
At 35, I was like India,
hot, relaxed
and convinced of my soul's innate music.
Then 40 hit me: BAM!
And there I was, a woman like France, gently aging
but still a desirable place to visit.
At 50, can you believe it, I was like Great Britain,
with a glorious past as a conqueror.
Now I'm 60, a woman like Yugoslavia,
who has lost the war and is haunted by her mistakes.
In May, I'll be 61,
a woman like Russia,
very wide with borders rarely patrolled.
And at 70, I hope to be like Tibet,
wildly beautiful with a mysterious past and the wisdom of all ages.

I lost my innocence the day my mother died. I was 25 years old.

Though my mother was never around much.

Growing up, I watched the best and the brightest, then developed an inferiority complex.

It's the perfect people I worship, bright, smart, sexy, funny, like my husband Roy. I trust them to define my boundaries, since they are so perfect.

I want truth serum in my tea. To help me know what is right and what is wrong. Every day, I throw out a little more rope, hoping that someday I'll lasso the truth.

Routine strangles me. The same. The same. Like a rope around my neck.

The rope popped open the scar from my brain surgeries. A gigantic 12-inch scar, hidden beneath my highlights. I'm different now.

To Roy, the mightiest of my G-ds, I say, "I like you differently now. Love you differently. I once liked your attention to detail, your belief in right and wrong."

I have been asked to be part of a fund-raising project. The title is "Right Knows No Boundaries." I am having a big problem with the title. Right does have boundaries to me.

There it is. The same, the same, the same. Those people on pedestals. They had boundaries. But I removed them, hungry as I was for praise.

They were G-ds, my G-ds. They were different, brilliant, original.

Oh well, to be honest, I have never known what was right.

Kindness, hugs, and smiles have been my guideposts for most of my life.

Roy said a few weeks ago, "There are no right or wrong answers." G-ddamit. There goes my innocence again.

My belief system blown apart. What do I believe?

I always thought that there was someone who had the answer, the complete understanding of right and wrong.

Do unto others as you would do unto yourself.

I never knew what was right, once my mother was gone.

I didn't know how to fight. To take flight. To take flight. Only to take flight.

These days, I fly.

I cry. I can't stop crying. Roy, did you want me to stay the same?

If only I had stayed the same. I would have liked you the same.

Loved you the same.

And the problems would be the same old ones I have always understood.

The same.

Boring.

"Love has no boundaries." Right has boundaries. Wrong has boundaries. But love has no boundaries, even with brain cancer.

My brain is handcuffed to a chair.
My heart is laid out on a table.
I have a permit to carry milk.
I am an art dealer.
Inside the car the police radio squawks to attention.
Still alive, I am supposed to have a honeymoon.
I scan the crowd as it moves past me.

My life keeps changing. I have found out I am pregnant with twins, a diptych. One embryo grows in my heart, the other in my brain. My womb is empty and dark. My docs, the GYN and my OB, say that the only thing I can be sure of at 60 is that my body will keep changing. I don't remember anything else they said except how to fix my womb: "Use it or lose it!" I read as many books as I can, but my comprehension of fact is missing. I require easy statements.

Gosh, G-d, how do I begin to understand all the things my family and friends are trying to tell me? Such good advice, too.

Or is it old wives' tales? I ask myself, who wags my tail? Who then, do I turn to for information? The Internet? I like the encyclopedia better because I can turn the pages and touch a rough leather cover while sitting in a rocking chair to read. I can control the light behind me, high or low.

In information theory, quantities are measured in units of information called bytes. It does have an "e" at the end. Gosh, the twin growing in my brain is going crazy. Sadie uses her veins to color her skin red so she will be known for her courage. I can feel her rocking back and forth in my head when I walk. Her knees are pulled up to her chest. The doctor showed me on the ultrasound. "Be careful of sunlight," he said. "You may be getting infrared rays, often called heat rays, resembling light rays. They can't be seen by the human eye."

Any object, such as a yellow rocking chair, gives off an infrared ray in relation to its temperature. The doctor told me that after I found out the baby growing in my brain is a girl. The one in my heart is a male. So I wear a sequined pink and blue baseball cap when I walk.

I will now have three daughters and soon a son. I think it is time for me to find out about males. All I know about them are the things I learned from Roy and all those guys who broke my heart: Ben, Jimmy, and Tricky Dickey. I am thrilled that the boy is growing in my heart. I will name him Sam, after my father. I will give birth to a boy who will teach me to understand the differences between the sexes. He will create an Initial Teaching Alphabet (I.T.A.) as a writing system. The I. T. A. is not intended to replace the traditional alphabet, but merely to ease my problems in learning to read and to comprehend change.

The fetus in my brain seems to be busting with independence. That's a girl for you. But the boy pushing his dick into my heart is having a harder time. I received an email from his lawyer. Here is what it said:

Dear Mom,

 This email serves as an injunction. I will soon be your son, Sam. I heard about you from my sister, Sadie, who is growing a few notches above me. She seems to be ahead of me. Mom, you must understand how important this injunction is. I want you to restore your mind to its former self: Your kindness, the pressure you feel to be a peacemaker, to multitask, and your ability to write with or without a voice. Mom, this is my voice. Open your mind to what I'm saying, it is MAN-datory. Step up to the plate, Mom! Get back your alertness and comprehension. You are too much of a free spirit, Mom. When you color . . . just stay on the page within the lines in the coloring book. Follow the rules. Get it together, Mom. This is not nonsense. "Injunctions have been known to stop Labor and cause a miscarriage."

Garfield, Katz, Canter, Rabbi & Goldstein
for soon-to-be-born Sam Rice Kaufman

Dear Sam,

 I made a party for your sister, Jennifer, who turned 35 on August 9th. I tried to get back to who I used to be by cooking lasagna for 18 people, multitasking perfectly, freezing it all ahead of time. I put the garlic bread in the freezer, next to two platters of chicken, meat and mushroom lasagna. My mind was alert enough to design several bouquets for the buffet tables. It was a beautiful sunny Sunday. Sam, I did all this by planning ahead, by taking a nap before the guests arrived, preparing the meal two days ahead of time, and thinking through all that was required. Two hours into the party I couldn't have been more proud. I felt G-d's light shining down on me. The mood and moon were perfect! Then, Sam, my sister-in-law said, "My, my Judi, you look tired. Go take a nap!" I said to her, "Please don't say that to me. I'm not tired." And she started to cry. So, see Sam, I need to be me, whoever I change into. I ripped up your injunction and went to the dining room and looked at the flower arrangements. I'm fine just the way I am. I welcome you into my world, when you are ready to be open to change.

Love, Mom

Lying awake in my king-size bed, I pause before getting up. The blinds are open. Sun seeps in. A new life grows inside my brain. Every morning I am in the dark. Confused. A different kind of morning sickness. I don't have a clue about pregnancy, since I have never been pregnant. I think G-d gave me brain cancer as a way to understand the physical and emotional changes in a woman. I am a different kind of mammal. I find out from other brain cancer survivors that gestation varies among different animals.

I have finally become a fetus. After a year I have recognizable human features. During those first months of recovery I had morning sickness. Nausea. Vomiting. Vertigo. I gained weight. My pants were hard to zip up.

A pregnant woman should have regular medical care during pregnancy. No problem. I have several physicians who advise me on what I can do about my lockjaw. I have difficulty opening and closing my mouth and I continually bite my tongue or the sides of my cheeks.

I have found the key to unlock my jaw. I bake dark chocolate sugar cookies for Roy. I frost them with yellow frosting to bring us back to light. I buy Baccarat crystal champagne goblets. I serve sparkling water in them at breakfast. They hold back nausea.

When my water breaks, I will invite my entire birthing group to drink my brain fluid in the crystal goblets.

Swollen feet, clumsy movement, aching back and indigestion, fear of the future.

During pregnancy a woman may feel increased depression or contentment.

I know them both.

Depression is particularly bad when I don't pace myself or when Roy looks depressed or disappointed in me. His lips turn down. He doesn't look at me. When I haven't cooked dinner for a few nights, it is especially depressing for him. When I don't feel safe to drive, I feel depressed. My friend said, "Your pregnancy would go much better if you would slow down your speech."

I told him that my doctors told me that my speech is as good as it is going to get. If it isn't perfect, it will merely remind people that I have had two miscarriages.

Increased contentment has been one of the benefits of pregnancy. On a good day, when I get enough sleep, I remember I am growing a new life.

I haven't given up living. I continue to learn how to avoid another miscarriage.

High blood pressure. Swollen ankles. Seizures. I try particularly hard not to miscarry. I walk carefully down a flight of stairs with the laundry or a box of beads to make into a necklace. The one I am working on now is made of pink square beads with letters on them. My baby's going to be a girl. I am going to name her SADIE, after my mother who died when I was 25.

I am a new woman. I am about to be a new kind of mother. I want to learn to be a better story teller, like my own mother. But I am exhausted when I try to talk or read. I have observed myself. When I talk for five minutes on the phone, I feel like I have been walking fast for 30 minutes. Sweating. Unable to breathe. My low blood pressure goes sky high. Before brain cancer I had energy and was a cheerful mother to my two daughters. From the minute I brought Jennifer home at two months I read to her in a yellow rocker.

Suzy came to live with us at two years, two months. I tried to read to her, but she wasn't interested. It wasn't until she was five that we found out she was hearing impaired. That is why she would turn my face toward her when I tried to talk to her. She was learning to read my lips. Still does. I turn people's faces toward me when I enter a room. For some reason people stare at me. I asked my psychiatrist about it.

"Yes!" he said, "people can see there is something different about you." I am not sure what they see. Am I getting fat, or is my mouth out of sync with my words?

I can't seem to get this new digital world. I must be an analog. Not pregnant. If I want to keep my new baby, not miscarry, I have to buy an adapter so I can plug my head into a battery. I will be ever-ready to grow and feed my baby. If I want to feel this new life, I must withstand the pain and prick of people. Take in the things that matter. The kicking of a new baby, the heartbeat, the rolling movement and the hiccups.

How about those eyes on the playing field of the ocean? Roy and I began to explore our history the day we brought Jennifer home. First we discovered her seashore, her skin, her small feet, her hands and her head. Year by year we saw that she was substantial, real, her left foot, her left hand, her head, all solid. Nothing sank, mirage-like, out of sight when you looked directly at it. Can you imagine this little blue-eyed beauty was sitting up at six months old? We went to Yamato's for a Japanese feast. Sitting in her high chair under the lanterns in a dark booth, her feet hung into the barrel below. We put clams, mussels and seaweeds on the table for tasting. This *shayna punim* picked up the clam shells and the pointed mussel shells. Her tiny tongue like a raft or small fishing boat swam over the shells.

Before Roy and I had dipped our sushi into the soy sauce and wasabi, Jennifer had dug the clam and muscle out of the shell.

Roy and I were fascinated. I was a little jealous. I knew at that moment there would be no stopping her. She has a vision all her own.

Jennifer, I whispered. *Do not compete with me, my Muffin. Just be yourself. Different, unusual, deep as the Pacific ocean. I'll be your mommy. I'll be myself. Whoever that is.*

Do you hear those waves? Those waves are your waves. Your ocean. They break against the shore, which is me, your mother. Don't worry. Let them come. I'm strong. I can stand it. Let them come forever—blue mysterious waves.

"Here, Kitty, Kitty," I called out as I walked into my walk-in closet. I am wondering what I should wear to go on my cat walk at 9:00 with my friend Doris. We have been walking, talking, and being cats for 25 years. It is chilly today. I know I want to feel thin. I put on my Nike Spandex tights; they were too tight until this week, and my hunter green sweatshirt I designed for myself 10 years ago. It says, "Anything is possible with good food, friends and family." After all, in two weeks I am supposed to be the mother of the bride. I am patching myself together to be ready.

But what, I wonder, does "Mother of the Bride" mean?

I feel like a cat in a hat. Who knows what magic I will have to pull off? I have to talk clearly and remember names for many hours. Talking requires more and more magic these days. A sentence from a fellow brain cancer survivor oozes through my brain. "I feel like there is another person in my brain." But me, I feel like there are seven portraits of me in my mind. I can't find the mother of the bride there, and when I do find it, I can't hang on to it.

Here are the seven portraits of me in my mind:
1) The Grand Chocolate Pizza Lady;
2) The Woman who started Etiquette International;
3) The Art of the Brain Founder;
4) American Jewish Committee VP Spreading Tolerance;
5) Wife;
6) Mother of two girls;
7) The mother of the bride.

But most of all, I want to be thin. I feel heavy with the chore of staying focused for 14 days. I put Pizza Protocol, AJC and AOB in their own covered boxes. I don't want to be selfish for this next 14 days. I cancelled my appointment with Cat for my physical and occupational therapy tomorrow. Tomorrow is about seating our guests. Not about me feeling good. Good enough to be a mother of the bride. Cat sounded kind of upset about me canceling a day ahead. I care about how she feels. Without Cat I would never have felt good enough to be the Mother of the Bride.

Judi, you are doing it again. Pull your claws in. Put all your responsibilities in their own boxes or in a book, like a journal. Just do what is right for Jennifer and Vlad.

I catch myself out of my cage.

I am under "S" for selfish in Webster's.

The chocolate pizza lady is in a triangular box.

My etiquette international and protocol are retired. Jennifer calls me this morning. "Mom, how do I address a thank-you note when the Rabbi and his wife are both doctors?"

Can't seem to mind my manners.

I remember the day we picked up Jennifer from the Adoption Agency. I went to pick up Roy. I was early. Roy was late. Roy is never late. I am always a little bit late. I remember Roy's left hand shaking when I tried to hold it with my right hand.

Jennifer was a late walker. She has never done things quickly. You see this is my first daughter to be married. She is 35.

I have wanted to be a mother since I was five. I would dress my cat in a baby outfit. I called my first dog "Baby." When I was 10, I went across the street to Mrs. Kanoke's house. She told me that she was Catholic and had only been able to conceive one child. She became a foster mother. From her, I learned all about fostering love. I was fearless at 10. I had only hand-me-downs to wear. They belonged to my sister, who was seven years older than I. I taught myself how to make her clothes look like art. I taught myself how to sew. I wore hats because I didn't know how to fix my hair.

Jennifer took a long time to pick the right man. I think she chose Vlad because he makes her laugh and feel calm. Roy and I don't laugh much. We didn't grow up with laughter. Our immigrant parents were doing all they could to survive in those post-World War II days.

Pay their bills.

Hide their Jewishness.

Educate their children.

Here I am reassuring myself that I am good enough to be the mother of the bride. Vlad and Jennifer, there are no boundaries for their beautiful brains. Love knows no boundaries.

I think most of my friends caught the drift of my learning to laugh again. My "Ha Ha's." The truth is, I never knew how to laugh. I wasn't learning to laugh again, I was learning to laugh in the first place. "Ha Ha Ha Ha Ha."

All the mother of the bride has to do is laugh with Jennifer and Vlad.

All I have to do is laugh, ha, ha, ha.

I start my morning off half-cocked, bellied up to the rosewood bar at the Focal Point on Rodeo Drive, 90210.

I speak slowly and clearly to the bartender, "I don't know what I mean by a cliché, I screwed up."

The bar is dancing with men in the A.M. and I begin moving down the bar, my eyes turned towards the glory.

The Glory I have seen, the cumming, of the Lord.

I linger there and here. I feel bare until my eyes sit on his highballs.

My favorite cliché is "Go Fuck Yourself," and sticks in my brain under my breath.

Gosh, G-d, Jesus Christ, Judi, it is time for you to have a time out and mend your fences and watch your p's and q's.

The time is right to write a book called *Judi-isms for the Brain-Injured* by mois, Judi Kaufman.

A cliché that cuts to the core of religion.

If you don't like it done to you, then don't do it to your friends, hmm?

Love thy neighbor as you love yourself?

Love makes the world go 'round, and life is just a bunch of cherries, I mean a bowl of cherries.

A tisket, a tasket, I want to be buried in a big red casket.

A tisket, a tasket, no please or pretty please, hear me loud and clear, "I want
    to be buried in a big red casket."
"Not blue, just a red pine box, like an orthodox Jew."
I will become a courageous Jew once the red paint is splashed on.
My friend's poor mom didn't get her last words and testament
    before she died.
Another friend said the owner of the same cemetery, Mt Sinai, said to her,
"You must be very secure, without an ounce of Jewish guilt, to leave your
    poor old mother in a pine box to rot."
Hey, you out there, don't you dare upgrade my casket! I want a pine box
and I am leaving three cans of red lacquer and a big fat paint brush with
    which to paint it.
I leave them with my two lawyers, Bruce and Barbara, in my vault with my
    last will and testament.
Read my last will and testament now and leave me alone when I am ready
    to die. I might not want to talk about it then.
Right before my last brain surgery I wrote my living will.
I wrote it in poetry and gave it to Bruce and Barbara on May 9th, my
    birthday, 2003.

2005 has arrived
and this last year was far and away my best year.
I bought what perfect people buy at Neiman Marcus,
especially the gifts they offer in the *Christmas Catalog.*
So what if they're wrapped in beige ribbon
garnished with a silver butterfly and a collector's picture frame?
Their biggest seller this year, top of the list, were framed
clichés by Donald Trump.
The categories include, "Parties, Christmas, Weddings and Bat Mitzvahs.
Funerals, Film Premieres, Flirting and Friendship."
Most of the people I know bought them.
The one I kept hearing the most, especially, after my daughter's wedding,
was "The room was so filled with love."
The clichés, which sold for $50,000 in a solid gold frame,
were reduced to half-price at Neiman Marcus's "Last call."
K-mart and Target have copies of the real deal,
solid brass framed clichés, two for five bucks!
I used to hate clichés; now they make my life easier.
I'm having a hard enough time talking.
I call myself a lymph, I walk with a lisp.
And if I try hard enough,
I'll learn the clichés, I'll know what to say
in any situation.
Finally, I believe in something, frisbeetarianism, which is when you die,
      your Soul flies up onto the roof and gets stuck there.

I am a fraud. For five years I said I had brain cancer. Not just a tumor. A malignant brain tumor. I had surgery to remove the golden ball from my head. On November 8, 1997. They gave me five years to survive. I got the five years. But shortly after that I started to have seizures every few months. So I had another brain surgery to remove another malignant brain tumor. I survived but I stopped cooking. So just the other night, I made a beautiful dinner party for our friends.

Shrying in Santa Fe and Sudan.
I don't want to scream.
Shrying.
I don't accomplish anything when I scream at people.
Especially standing beneath the sun roof,
in the light of my lovers and friends.
In the political light of presidents, family, sisters and brothers.
Then I would have sold out to a system.
A system that screams at sadness.
A system that listens through death's ears to strangled, starving souls.
Shrying and screaming.
At presidents who lie
And starve souls in Sudan.
People are sitting ducks.
I have gone lame; I am a sitting duck and I have lost my scream.

I got into CAL—
The University of California at Berkeley.
I got in on my ability to get A's.
My parents,
their faces graded me a B-.
They were afraid I would love orgies.

It is a moonlit night and my mind is not made up.
It is made of loud noises from back in the day.
Love is loud and sweaty sometimes, it makes me die.
Shut-up, love from back in the day
when Clint called me "Jude the Prude from Pasadena."
My first secret passion and petting still screams into my ear.
I met Matt on a hot Monday and he was hot with terror.
He has a non-malignant brain tumor.
Matt thinks I'm hot because I have survived brain cancer.
I get lots of credit for surviving brain cancer.
And I have to admit,
There is something sexy about brain cancer, isn't there?

The bottle sits before me on the bar.
Dark beer from Utah.
It's called Polygamy Porter.
The label says, "Why have just one?"
Picture one man
With seven women, legs spread wide.
As my Jewish grandmother would say, *"Vy haf just von?"*
When I was 16, I wanted to be an LDS.
A Latter-Day Saint.
I want to be Mormon, I screamed.
Now I know why.
It's this bottle, this label.
The bottle is hard,
With a golden tip.
In the light from the window,
It looks like a golden cock.
I drink it down in one swig.
The bartender comes over.
"Gimme another," I say.
"Why have just one?"

My husband Roy said to me, "I read that a woman uses twice as many
    words as a man during a conversation."
"That's because a woman has to tell a man everything twice," I said.
"What?" said Roy.
"I am alone and lonely," I said, in my darkest voice
"Why?" he asked.
A pillar of steam rose slowly through the grate of my scar.
The steam undulated across the floor of my brain before it climbed into the
    chilly air.
I tapped my index nail on the coffee table.
My once beautiful pair of legs planted in three-inch black high heels sliced
    through the air towards him and stopped.
"Why do you think I had a non-malignant brain tumor?" I said.
"What? What are you talking about?"
"I had a malignant brain tumor in 1997 and in 2002, two golf balls removed
    from my brain, just like that."
Two nine-hour surgeries later.
"I don't know what you are talking about, Judi."
"What are you talking about, Roy?"
"What are YOU talking about? You had an ordinary tumor, not a
    malignant tumor?"
"Really, Roy, so all the things we have been doing these last seven years, to
    help me walk, talk, tell time and have sex has been a big fraud?
I screamed, "I still have a malignant tumor!
Brain cancer never goes into remission.
Face it. I have."
"I'll get back to you tomorrow, Judi."

Six months ago I decided to get my hair scissors sharpened.
I have had my scissors since I was seven and wore straight bangs.
I used them for years to cut my bangs when I wore my hair
      in a bob, then a flip.
I was a brunette then, in 1963. Now it's 2005
      and I am probably almost gray.
My highlights hide a multitude of sins, including my brain cancer scars.
Those old hair scissors, they have cut away my guilt and shame
As well as hundreds of tags off all the clothes I have bought for the last 30
      years.
Before that, I couldn't afford Barney's.
I was stuck in junior high school hand-me-downs, so I would sew and sew
      until I had seven outfits, one for each day of the week.
Then I became very popular.
When Jennifer was three months old, I gave her her first haircut.
She was sitting up at three months old.
I didn't want her huge head of hair to cover her eyes.
Her blue eyes brought people closer to us.
I took a strip of Scotch tape to hold down her wet hair
      mixed with a little gel.
Roy said, "Are you sure you know what you are doing?"
He still asks me that when he see me take out my scissors.

I have gone south of my brain stem.
South of my center.
I am crossing over the border.
People say I don't make sense.
They say I am becoming a sexpot,
That my soup discharges into my days.

The light of my hills and the darkness of my valleys, wow!
I diminished myself and harmed others, wow!
I pretended emotions I did not feel until now, wow!
I used the sins of others to excuse my own, wow!
I protected my ego until I started growing brain cancer, wow.
I let my sometimes pretty face and happy smile hide me, wow!
My daily rounds and cares prevented me from going inward.
Wow, my inward trek!
Wow, I am stumbling over the edge of life in Carmel.
G-d, this is not the time for me to be *KASH-EL OR-EF*
      (a stiff-necked person).
I number my days while wishing for wisdom, wow.
I waited till now
To commit to my marriage, wow!
So Roy and I lie side by side together,
No longer waiting,
no longer pretending.
Wow.

I have been in the dark for so many months, feeling nothing.
Light and laughter sit by my side like atrophied limbs.
Like shadows of my personal war.
Terrorism is part of all of our lives now.
So I sit down with my Rabbi and friend, Uri Herscher.
"How do I tie my personal experience and my passion, into this day of my
    Bat Mitzvah?" I ask him.
Uri begins with a tough question (as a Jew usually does).
"Judi, do you know why all Jewish holidays begin at nightfall?"
"No, Uri, I don't."
He takes out the Old Testament, a book that belongs to all of us.
He reads me the first paragraph from Genesis.
In the beginning G-d created the heaven and earth.
The earth was a formless void.
Darkness covered the face of the waters.
Then G-d said, "Let there be light."
And G-d saw that light was good.
And G-d separated the light from the darkness.
G-d called the light Day and the darkness Night.
And there was evening, and there was morning, the first day.
Uri said, "Before you can see the dawn of the day you have to experience
    darkness…and then light so you can see the sun rise and the sun set.
    G-d's first deed was light."
So we gathered together for a celebration.
Life is a collaboration.
We came together to watch the light come forth.
I'm on my way.
But I'm still confused.
Where is my laughter?
I don't want to be detached.
Once again I seek out a friend for some wisdom and collaboration.
I ask my writing mentor, Jack Grapes, how to laugh.
He reminds me to go to my darkness where I will find my light.
"Don't be afraid," he says, "just make a fool of yourself."
He tells me to begin by saying "Ha" once.
Then "ha-ha."

Then "ha ha ha."

"Don't muffle your laughter, just say 'Ha ha ha ha,' four times."

Now I'm laughing at myself.

I am 60!

Today is my Bat Mitzvah!

People started laughing when I started planning it.

Ha

Ha Ha

Ha Ha Ha

Ha Ha Ha Ha

Ha Ha Ha Ha Ha

"You're not a child," they said.

"Sorry, I am a child!

Somehow I got to 60."

They told me that a Bat Mitzvah was supposed to be about me.

"Ha Ha HA."

Now I'm really laughing,

"Ha Ha Ha Ha Ha!"

"No way!"

My Bat Mitzvah is going to be about my family, my friends, the Art of My Brain, and you and me.

Me, as an American Jew, and you with whatever beliefs you hold close.

It is a unique honor to share this day with you.

Today, I want to be surrounded by you, my family and friends,

I want to laugh with you so that there may be light.

I want to share a meal with you, for as you know, food has always been my muse.

We will observe tolerance together, share differences and break bread together.

There's nothing to laugh at here: this is BIG stuff.

People laughed at me when I wrote about my sex life.

Our sex life.

The title of my second book was "Passions and Shadows, the Lights of Brain Cancer."

But Roy was proud of me—he never laughed.

Instead he said, "I love your red lips, your red nails and your red courage."

Jennifer and Suzy said, "Mom, Daddy's right!"

So I am not so sane.

I practice laughing, I'm just a little left-of-center.

Ha!

Ha ha!

I dream of about finding a way to bring people closer
    together through collaboration.

America is a world of differences.

Still, can't we sit down together for tea and a nosh?

Every country, every culture has its own style of bread.

I love them all. Why limit ourselves to breaking only one style
    of bread together?

The French say *Bonjour* to their baguettes.

The Mid-Westerners say *Hey* to their white bread.

The Italians say *Mama Mia* to their focaccio.

The Latinos say *Buenas Tardes* to their hand-made tortillas.

The Chinese say *Nee How* to their buns.

The Russians say *Privyot* to their dark Pumpernickel.

The Germans say *Guten Tag* to their mandelbroit.

So G-d Bless bread and all its possibilities.

I ask you now to laugh with me.

Laugh once:

Ha

Ha, ha.

Ha, ha, ha.

Thank you for adding a little more light to this already beautiful room.

Here I am, at 60, speaking and laughing.

I am happy!

I am alive!

I can laugh again!

But only because of your support and love, your collaboration and wisdom.

So indulge me, my family and friends.

I have a new brain!

That's what makes it so hard to count my "Ha-Ha's."

But big deal.

"I like you just the way you are!"

And I hope you like me just as I am.

So I speak funny.

Don't be scared of my lisps and slurs.

We are family, we are friends.

Together we are a miracle.
We laugh!
We cry!
We are all alive, together,
at this moment in time,
helping each other to feel more whole.
So, ha, ha to the fear!
Ha, ha to the sadness!
Ha, ha to the afflictions of the mouth and the tongue!
Ha, ha to the history of consolation and regret!
Ha, ha to passion and shadow, cakes and ale.
Ha ha ha ha ha ha ha ha ha ha!
Thank you Roy, my main collaborator, and Jennifer, Suzy,
        family and friends.
Thank you, Rabbis.
Thank you, Cantor.
Let us break bread together, in celebration of this day, this moment.
Ha!

I love men's beards because
They show off the design of their pubic hair.
I would love to run my hands over their heads
and their hearts.
Thick and grey is best.
It brings out my secrets.

Yesterday, another comrade died
of brain cancer.
His name was Robert.
He signed seven cards before he died.
His mother drove down from Modesto
to make sure I got one of them.

Meshugass—Mad, *Meshuga*—Crazy
Meshugeit ahf toit!—Crazy as a loon.
Insane about hair
I am disgusted when I find hair in my food.
Meshugena—A mad, crazy, insane woman.
A *shid-a-ryne*—a little of this and a lot of that.

For most of my life.
Friends and family thought I was a phony.
Not real, too nice!
Then I got brain cancer.
There is nothing phony about my scar:
14 inches hidden beneath a big plastic clip.

Gossip

We never said goodbye.
This time we will be bigger.
Braver, brainier.
Has there ever been such a moment,
such an opportunity?
Whispered conversation in the bathroom,
like a brain has to tell its story.
So, there are memories.
Moments of my soul.
Something that lasts
like a legacy but simpler,
easier, as casual as gossip.

I have always loved heroes. My heroes are leaders, like Ben Franklin.
Ben helped me to find my brain, bravery, my balls.
I play with my balls these days, but I am confused by my heroes.
Where in my wiring did my roots of truth come from?
I am sitting at Starbucks, in Beverly Hills on Beverly Drive.
Today in this new time, wired, windless, the traffic steals away my breath.
My breath is in the gas tank with gallons of cell phones.
Lots of phones with dials, Pasadena kind of phones, party lines.
A gorgeous man walks by, I know him, and he used to be my hero.
The kind I would dream about, like Ben, but his bifocals were gone.
I watched him take them off when he saw me;
     he threw them at the gas tank.
He pretended he didn't see me; he was the man
     who always wanted to know.
I am a committee of confusion; Ben and boys have been confused by me.
Back in my day in Pasadena, I was blowing in the Sycamore wind.
I am my own hero, surviving two brain cancer surgeries,
under the guidance of my deaf heart.

Since the day I met her,
She has craved power and men,
trying to get into all the players' pants.
Including mine and those of the other women.
She did it because she could.
Her power lies in her words.
"I am confused,"
she says, and it's true,
she is confused, and so beautiful
because of it.

Imagine this, I came out of the oven clapping.
Once I figured out how to measure,
I have been much more interested in the hue of food.
You know what I mean,
take Mandelbroit for example,
hey babe out there, Jewish biscotti.
It is best when it is dark with a lot of chocolate.
And crispy or darker when it comes out of the womb.
For slicing and light enough in the room.
So that the whole family can smell a light touch of cinnamon.
If their brains are still filled with light gray matter.
The gray matter comes from the gluten in the flour.
Just take a handful of flour and wash it under the faucet,
      about eight minutes.
In life and in cooking, timing is everything!
Eventually you will end up with a mass of gray matter.
I will teach you to cook both light and dark.

I love doing the dirty work.
Even if he is a *Shaigitz* with a *petseleh*.
A wild Jewish boy with a little penis and little hair.
Appearing to offer passion, food and wine
Having a love affair with life.
Those guys surrender to secrets.

My yoga teacher just arrived.
She rings the front door like a Christmas bell.
I lead her to my guest house for a session.
I am pouting.
I mean my pussy is pouting.
My lips are turned down.
I am doing yoga.
I forgot to put on my leggings.
My legs stretch out in the outfield.
I've got my head under my spread legs.
I look up and see that someone has cut off my balls.
I stretch my arms above my head
Maybe my brain is hiding my missing balls.
I'm scarred from head to toe.
Scars are my tattoos for my once brave soul.
I saw my balls bounce away.
Amnesia has set in.
I don't remember when that bounce first happened.
Lost years.
My tender testicles were once filled with testosterone.
To test my brain.
My doctor was shocked to see my balls bounce away.
He has amnesia too.
He forgot he took out two golf balls.
He should have written that down on my chart.
My courage chart.
He never even said, "I'm sorry!"
But we know that docs never say, "I'm sorry."
Most have lost their balls too.

Prick the Matzoh with a fork.
This pricking keeps giant bubbles from forming.
My Matzoh is round, not square.
Transfer to baking sheet, and bake at 475° for six to eight minutes.
Keep an eye on it, it may burn; remove and wrap tightly.
Skip the whole damn thing, make Matzoh balls instead.

When his face became paralyzed, Nanai cooked *Sinigang* soup.

Tatai could not swallow or chew.

Cancer made them cut away his jaw, Nanai knew her job.

She would sew soup and cover and steam it with a patchwork.

Even when his records were broken,

she could make him laugh and dance with the music.

This Filipino woman cooked like a Jew, a *shid-a-ryne*.

Chicken Soup with white and dark fish.

The garnish was a bouquet of orchids from Hawaii.

Nanai grew *jabong* (grapefruit), mango, and banana trees in her yard, along
    with the orchids.

Nanai named every piece of fruit after her friends.

When, she found herself on a Hoyer lift, she couldn't move
    and needed help.

Her life was dark, she wanted to die.

One day she was up in the air, she sang

"Fly Me to the Moon."

I want to see Tatai.

Brian is all about appearances.
When I touch his arm, he flexes his muscles.
"Judi, you look so pretty, lighter and brighter."
"What would you have looked like after two brain cancer surgeries?" I said.
Not a pretty comeback.
More confident now,
I can be ugly, nasty and truthful.

His body isn't even cold yet.
His friends from the hood are already calling him names.
His good name is forsaken.
Shaking, shivering sentences that don't belong in an obituary.
Odd, impeccable and gay, they implied.
His sons heard all of it; they were sobbing their eyes out.
I stood up and said, "At least he knew how to love."

Snow and ashes.
Light and dark.
I try to see the light,
but I need yellow glasses.
I always seem to wear
sunglasses so I see black.
I can't undress the need to be a deb.
White picket fences I tried to open.
Brunette and gray beneath my light streaks.
Phony color.
In a timeless realm.
I have tried to be a graceful debutante,
a loving debutante,
in my flowing white ball gown.
I should be wearing a little black dress,
with stains of bittersweet chocolate.
They can barely be seen.
I sew on ruffles of
Sweet white chocolate
under moon light.
Yes is the light.
No is the dark.
Stop he says.
Now I say, stop.
Maybe I am too late for light.
Stand up and say what you want.
But he hears dark.
I ask for truth.
Delete the truth, he asks me.
He wrote his eulogy.
I looked at it,
then he told me to delete it.
I said yes instead of no.
I could have just hidden it.
It is I who is dark.
Help me, I can not find my light.

I am weak.
I have always been weak.
I just wanted to believe
in light
His light.

My Rabbi
once again spoke to me of life.
He called me on Yom Kippur,
before sunset on the Day of Atonement.
I have kept the message now for several weeks.
It is still there.
On that day when G-d decides,
who will live and who will die?
Doing great deeds will keep the gate open.
When I wake up dark and vulnerable,
I do bad deeds.
I say to myself, every day,
today is a day to do great deeds.
By the light of the day.
The time G-d starts a new day
is the time to do a good deed.
The Rabbi said the gate is always open.
When I forget and do a dark deed,
I remember and start my day over.
Even if the sun has set.
I can remove the darkness in my heart.
I scare away the scar tissue of darkness
by lighting one candle.
I call a sick friend.
I bake cookies in memory
of someone who has passed on.
Cooking for continuity.
I will teach kids again
how to cook for continuity,
how to light candles.
Deeds open doors to gardens,
And to goodness.

The 61-year-old woman that once was me.
The 92-year-old Filipino woman.
The 62-year-old female friend dying of lung and brain cancer.
The 82-year-old alcoholic writer.
The 32-year-old woman looking to get married and have a child.
The 30-year-old brain-injured woman.
The 37-year-old housekeeper that dances without a green card.
I can't stop caring about
The 22-year-old boy with the motorcycle.

I hate my Palm Pilot. Roy uses it to make sure I am safe, hot-syncing my calendar to his hard drive.

He came up with a system so he knows that I am OK.

With my Palm Pilot, in conjunction with my computer, Roy knows at any given moment where I am, what I am doing and with whom. He developed a simple system based on letters. R stands for Roy, J stands for Judi, and K stands for Kaufman.

RJK in caps stands for Roy and Judi together. I have to remember the alphabet, A through Z. I am fine when I say A, B, C, D, E, F, G, H, I, J and K.

After K I have to start all over again.

I can't remember what comes after K. "rjk" in small letters stands for me alone doing an activity as an independent woman.

So when I put something down on my calendar, first I have to find the right month, then the right day, then remember if it is for Roy and I to do together or if I will be doing it alone.

Alone.

What comes after K?

What comes after everything other than K?

Then I have to assign it to a time frame. Will it last an hour or two? How would I know? You never know how long things last.

My first birthday party lasted two hours. My 60th birthday, my Bat Mitzvah this year, lasted five hours. My first marriage is still lasting.

But you never know how long anything will last.

After K, anything is possible.

That's why I like spontaneity.

Time to take in the details, the colors, the way things feel. I don't want to be caught up in a schedule. Do this first. Do that now. Do this then. Save this for last.

Everything right on time. Nothing left to chance, nothing after K.

But everything good comes after K. My two daughters, Jennifer and Suzy.

Then I have to remember, does Roy want to go to an AJC, American Jewish Committee and plate dinner, or should I go alone?

Who will drive me there, who will pick me up?

There are so many questions, so much unanswered, so much undone.

I have to find a way to get Palming down to a science.

What the hell does Roy want?

For instance:

He goes to all of my doctor appointments with me, so that would mean RJK in caps in my Palm Pilot. Business events including luncheon dates, those occasions would be a little rjk so Roy knows he can't come.

Of course there's that brunch with Bunny Wasser and Howard Bernstein in Malibu, strictly social, not business.

But I see an uppercase RJK. I guess that means Roy wants to come. In lowercase rjk there's "thank you" notes to all my friends at Art of the Brain. I send those out by myself alone, after K.

I am not a geometry genius.
Infinite lines,
finite points,
proven assumptions,
give me a headache.
Postulates and theorems.
Congruent angles.
Parallel lines.
Self-evident axioms.
Obvious truths!
I flunked geometry.
You know Euclid's theory? That one and only one parallel to a given line
    can be drawn through a point external to a line?
Well, it can't be proven from his other postulates. It took them 20 centuries
    to discover that, but now the cat's out of the bag.
So now they've got Non-Euclidian Geometry. If something works, it's
    Something-idian. And if it doesn't work, it's Non-Something-idian.
After K.
Where you're alone.
Where all parallel lines meet.
Where anything can happen.
I know there's a way to connect the gaps.
Calendars are made up of squares. I have to get some other shapes on my
    calendar. Parallel lines. Hexagons. Triangles. Pentagons. Rectangles.
Diagonals running from corner to corner.
The collaboration of horizontal, vertical and diagonal lines which form
    landscapes and portraits.
These days I have to learn everything all over again. How many days in a
    week? Seven. That's not so bad. Imagine if there were 16.
You'd forget when Tuesday is coming, or Friday. But with seven, you
    know what to expect. On the seventh day, I get to rest without
    feeling guilty.
Then I come face to face with the month.
"How many days in a month?" I ask myself. I can't remember. So I make a
    fist.
A non-Euclidian geometrical figure. Square, triangle, fist.

Starting from my outside knuckle I begin with January. In the valley of my
knuckles is February.
I continue to the fourth knuckle and I start on the outside knuckle again.
All the knuckles have 31 days and the valleys have 30 days.
But leap year is easy for me.
I remember that February has 29 days instead of 28.
"30 days has my fist, knuckle valley and a twist.
All the rest have fingernails,
except for my thumb."

We're a long way from K, from geometry and parallel lines.

"Humpty Dumpty sat on a wall. Humpty Dumpty had a great fall. All the king's horses (and the king had lots of horses, believe me), and all the king's men (and there were lots of them), couldn't put Humpty Dumpty together again."

Roy is trying to put ME together again.

But I can't seem to remember it's the year we're in.

I am an egg that fell off the wall.

Roy uses the Palm Pilot as glue to put me back into one piece, but his glue blocks the light of my yolk.

I like the light shining through the cracked shells.

I am put together better now in a Non-Euclidian way.

I am hard-boiled, my skin sticks to me.

No matter how long I rinse myself in cold water, the shells will not come off. They're part of my thin skin.

I like being scrambled too.

There is no separation of white and yellow—just a more subtle relationship between the two.

I enjoy the chaos of life, the mixture of the many colors, the non-Euclidian merging of parallel lines and unproved assumptions.

If only I could teach Roy how to scramble eggs instead of using the Palm Pilot to divide my days into hexagons, pentagons, triangles and rectangles.

We would become two congruent circles enclosing uppercase RJK and lowercase rjk, both of them smack dab in the middle.

Printed in the United States
65775LVS00002B/1-339

9 780941 017800